30-Minute One-Pot Meals

Crockpot cookbook
For men

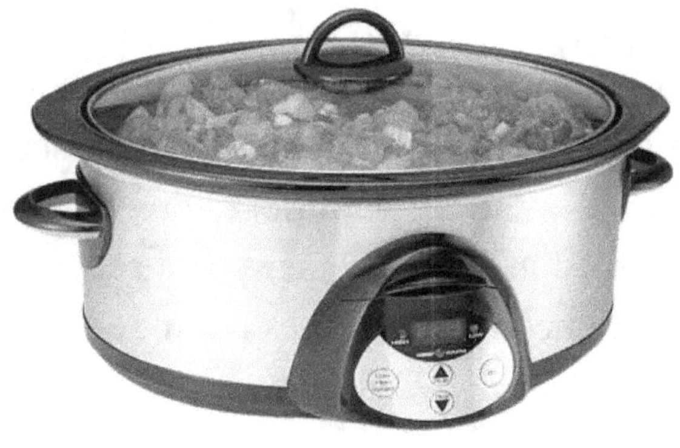

30 Tasty and Nourishing Slow Cooker Recipes for Busy Men

Vivian Greene

Table of contents

Introduction 6

Chapter 1 9

Hearty Soups and Stews......................... 9

Beef and Barley Stew......................... 9

Chicken Noodle Soup 11

Spicy Chili Con Carne 13

Chapter 2 15

Easy Weeknight Dinners...................... 15

Slow Cooker BBQ Pulled Pork 15

Garlic and Herb Roast Chicken 17

Sausage and Peppers 19

Chapter 3 21

Comforting Pasta and Grains 21

Creamy Mac and Cheese 21

Beefy Pasta Bolognese.................... 23

Mediterranean Quinoa Bowl............ 25

Chapter 4 27

Flavorful International Dishes 27

Chicken Tikka Masala 27

Mexican Beef Carnitas...................... 30

Thai Red Curry.................................. 32

Chapter 5 34

Healthy Vegetarian Options................. 34

Lentil and Vegetable Curry.............. 34

Ratatouille 36

Veggie-Packed Minestrone.............. 38

Chapter 6 40

Sweet Treats and Desserts 40

Slow Cooker Apple Crisp 40

Chocolate Lava Cake 42

Berry Bread Pudding....................... 44

More recipes to indulge.......................... 46

Chicken and Rice Casserole.............. 46

Vegetarian Chili 47

Lemon Garlic Chicken 48

Beef and Broccoli............................. 49

Creamy Mushroom and Spinach Pasta
.... 50

Crockpot Ratatouille 52

Teriyaki Turkey Meatballs................ 53

Mediterranean Quinoa Stew 54

Lemon Herb Salmon 55

BBQ Pulled Pork Sandwiches 56

Creamy Chicken Alfredo Pasta......... 57

Beef Burrito Bowls 59

Mediterranean Chicken with Olives and Artichokes 60

Crockpot Beef and Vegetable Curry . 61

Lemon Garlic Butter Shrimp 62

Turkey and Sweet Potato Chili 63

Hawaiian Pineapple Chicken 65

Creamy Mushroom Chicken.............. 66

Conclusion 68

Introduction

I've worked as a professional nutritionist who is committed to encouraging healthy eating, and I've met a lot of people who are looking for methods to fit nutritional meals into their busy schedules. My spouse, James, was notable among them not only as my life partner but also as the person whose culinary adventures served as inspiration for my cookbook.

Like many men juggling hectic schedules and demanding occupations, James often found himself prioritizing convenience over health. He followed a road where takeaway cartons and fast food wrappers were his usual companions due to his long work hours and packed schedule. Convenience overshadowed health—a sentiment shared by many in comparable situations.

Seeing his suffering inspired me to go out on a quest. I came to see that convenience didn't have to come at the expense of flavor or health. I introduced James to the benefits of slow cooking, using my knowledge of nutrition to make our meals more nutritional and easy.

Our kitchen's unsung hero quickly emerged as our crockpot. It simmered not only the ingredients but also James's newly discovered enthusiasm for cooking. It solved his time restrictions and allowed us to enjoy nutrient-dense, tasty, handmade meals.

This cookbook is more than simply a collection of recipes; it's a record of James's journey and a manual for those guys who, like him, like delectable meals without devoting long hours to the kitchen. These pages include a variety of recipes that are made to satisfy your palate and take care of your health, even if you have a hectic schedule.

With the care and skill of a nutritionist and the love of a wife who wants the best for her husband, each dish has been painstakingly created. These recipes, which range from robust stews to exotic treats, are not only very simple to make but also packed with all the vital nutrients your body needs.

I cordially welcome you to join me on this gastronomic journey, combining the ease of a crockpot with the knowledge of a nutritionist. Allow this cookbook to be your guide as you create meals that satisfy your palate and nourish your body while also fitting into your schedule.

Cheers to healthy, tasty food, even at the busiest times of life.

Chapter 1

Hearty Soups and Stews

Beef and Barley Stew

Ingredients:

1. 1 pound beef stew meat, cubed
2. 1 cup barley, rinsed
3. 4 cups beef broth
4. 1 onion, chopped
5. 3 carrots, sliced
6. 3 celery stalks, chopped
7. 2 cloves garlic, minced
8. 1 teaspoon dried thyme
9. Salt and pepper to taste

Instructions:

1. In a crockpot, combine beef, barley, beef broth, onion, carrots, celery, garlic, thyme, salt, and pepper.
2. Stir well to combine ingredients.

3. Cook on low for 7-8 hours or on high for 4-5 hours until beef is tender and barley is cooked through.
4. Adjust seasoning if needed and serve hot.

Nutrition per Serving (serving size - 1.5 cups):

- ❖ Calories: 320
- ❖ Total Fat: 8g
- ❖ Saturated Fat: 3g
- ❖ Cholesterol: 70mg
- ❖ Sodium: 680mg
- ❖ Total Carbohydrates: 34g
- ❖ Dietary Fiber: 7g
- ❖ Sugars: 4g
- ❖ Protein: 28g

Chicken Noodle Soup

Ingredients:

1. 2 boneless, skinless chicken breasts
2. 8 cups chicken broth
3. 2 carrots, sliced
4. 2 celery stalks, chopped
5. 1 onion, diced
6. 2 cloves garlic, minced
7. 1 teaspoon dried thyme
8. 2 cups egg noodles
9. Salt and pepper to taste
10. Fresh parsley for garnish (optional)

Instructions:

1. Place chicken breasts, chicken broth, carrots, celery, onion, garlic, and thyme in the crockpot.
2. Cook on low for 6-7 hours or on high for 3-4 hours until chicken is cooked through.
3. Remove chicken, shred it, and return it to the pot.

4. Add egg noodles to the crockpot, cooking for an additional 15-20 minutes until noodles are tender.
5. Season with salt and pepper, garnish with parsley if desired, and serve hot.

Nutrition per Serving (serving size - 1.5 cups):

- ❖ Calories: 240
- ❖ Total Fat: 4g
- ❖ Saturated Fat: 1g
- ❖ Cholesterol: 65mg
- ❖ Sodium: 780mg
- ❖ Total Carbohydrates: 20g
- ❖ Dietary Fiber: 2g
- ❖ Sugars: 3g
- ❖ Protein: 28g

Spicy Chili Con Carne

Ingredients:

1. 1 pound ground beef
2. 1 onion, chopped
3. 2 cloves garlic, minced
4. 1 bell pepper, diced
5. 1 can (14 oz) diced tomatoes
6. 1 can (14 oz) kidney beans, drained and rinsed
7. 2 tablespoons chili powder
8. 1 teaspoon cumin
9. 1 teaspoon paprika
10. Salt and pepper to taste

Instructions:

1. In a skillet, brown the ground beef with onion, garlic, and bell pepper until beef is cooked through. Drain excess fat.
2. Transfer the beef mixture to the crockpot. Add diced tomatoes, kidney beans, chili powder, cumin, paprika, salt, and pepper.
3. Stir well to combine ingredients.

4. Cook on low for 6-7 hours or on high for 3-4 hours.

5. Adjust seasoning if needed and serve hot.

Nutrition per Serving (serving size - 1 cup):

- ❖ Calories: 320
- ❖ Total Fat: 14g
- ❖ Saturated Fat: 6g
- ❖ Cholesterol: 60mg
- ❖ Sodium: 640mg
- ❖ Total Carbohydrates: 22g
- ❖ Dietary Fiber: 7g
- ❖ Sugars: 5g
- ❖ Protein: 25g

Chapter 2

Easy Weeknight Dinners

Slow Cooker BBQ Pulled Pork

Ingredients:

1. 2 lbs pork shoulder or pork butt, trimmed of excess fat
2. 1 cup barbecue sauce
3. ½ cup chicken or beef broth
4. 1 tablespoon brown sugar
5. 1 tablespoon Worcestershire sauce
6. 1 teaspoon smoked paprika
7. 1 teaspoon garlic powder
8. Salt and pepper to taste
9. Hamburger buns, for serving

Instructions:

1. In a bowl, mix together barbecue sauce, broth, brown sugar, Worcestershire sauce, smoked paprika, garlic powder, salt, and pepper.

2. Place the pork shoulder or pork butt in the slow cooker.
3. Pour the barbecue sauce mixture over the pork, ensuring it's evenly coated.
4. Cook on low for 8-10 hours or on high for 4-6 hours until the pork is tender and easily shreds with a fork.
5. Once done, shred the pork using two forks. Mix it with the remaining sauce in the slow cooker.
6. Serve the pulled pork on hamburger buns and enjoy!

Nutrition per Serving (pulled pork only, without bun):

- ❖ Calories: 250 kcal
- ❖ Protein: 25g
- ❖ Carbohydrates: 15g
- ❖ Fat: 10g
- ❖ Fiber: 1g
- ❖ Sugar: 12g

Garlic and Herb Roast Chicken

Ingredients:

1. 1 whole chicken (3-4 lbs), giblets removed
2. 4 cloves garlic, minced
3. 2 tablespoons fresh herbs (such as rosemary, thyme, or sage), chopped
4. 2 tablespoons olive oil
5. Salt and pepper to taste

Instructions:

1. Rinse the chicken and pat it dry with paper towels.
2. In a small bowl, mix together the minced garlic, chopped herbs, olive oil, salt, and pepper.
3. Rub the herb mixture all over the chicken, including under the skin and inside the cavity.
4. Place the chicken in the slow cooker.
5. Cook on low for 6-7 hours or on high for 3-4 hours until the chicken reaches an internal temperature of 165°F (74°C) in the thickest part.

6. Once done, let the chicken rest for 10-
   15 minutes before carving.

Nutrition per Serving (3 oz of cooked chicken, approximate):

- ❖ Calories: 180 kcal
- ❖ Protein: 25g
- ❖ Carbohydrates: 0g
- ❖ Fat: 8g
- ❖ Fiber: 0g
- ❖ Sugar: 0g

Sausage and Peppers

Ingredients:

1. 1 lb Italian sausage (sweet or spicy), sliced
2. 2 bell peppers (red, green, or yellow), sliced
3. 1 onion, sliced
4. 2 cloves garlic, minced
5. 1 can (14 oz) diced tomatoes, drained
6. 1 teaspoon Italian seasoning
7. Salt and pepper to taste
8. Fresh parsley, chopped (optional, for garnish)

Instructions:

1. In a skillet over medium heat, brown the sliced sausage until cooked through. Drain excess fat if needed.
2. Place the cooked sausage, sliced bell peppers, onion, minced garlic, diced tomatoes, Italian seasoning, salt, and pepper in the slow cooker.
3. Mix everything together until well combined.

4. Cook on low for 6-8 hours or on high for 3-4 hours.

5. Serve the sausage and peppers on its own or over cooked rice or pasta. Garnish with chopped parsley if desired.

Nutrition per Serving (approximate, without rice or pasta):

- ❖ Calories: 320 kcal
- ❖ Protein: 15g
- ❖ Carbohydrates: 10g
- ❖ Fat: 25g
- ❖ Fiber: 3g
- ❖ Sugar: 5g

Chapter 3

Comforting Pasta and Grains

Creamy Mac and Cheese

Ingredients:

1. 2 cups elbow macaroni
2. 2 cups shredded cheddar cheese
3. 1 cup milk
4. 1/4 cup unsalted butter
5. 1/4 cup all-purpose flour
6. 1/2 teaspoon salt
7. 1/2 teaspoon black pepper
8. Optional: breadcrumbs for topping

Instructions:

1. Cook the elbow macaroni according to package instructions until al dente. Drain and set aside.
2. In the crockpot, melt the butter over low heat. Add flour and whisk until smooth, cooking for 2 minutes.

3. Slowly pour in the milk while whisking continuously to avoid lumps.
4. Add shredded cheddar cheese, salt, and pepper, stirring until the cheese melts and the sauce thickens.
5. Add the cooked macaroni to the cheese sauce in the crockpot, stirring until well combined.
6. Optional: Sprinkle breadcrumbs on top for a crispy finish.
7. Cover and cook on low for 1-2 hours or until heated through.

Nutrition per Serving:

- ❖ Calories: 380
- ❖ Fat: 20g
- ❖ Carbohydrates: 30g
- ❖ Protein: 18g

Beefy Pasta Bolognese

Ingredients:

1. 1 pound ground beef
2. 1 onion, diced
3. 3 cloves garlic, minced
4. 1 can (28 ounces) crushed tomatoes
5. 1 teaspoon dried oregano
6. 1 teaspoon dried basil
7. Salt and pepper to taste
8. 2 cups pasta of your choice

Instructions:

1. In a skillet over medium heat, brown the ground beef until cooked through. Drain excess fat.
2. Transfer the cooked beef to the crockpot. Add diced onions, minced garlic, crushed tomatoes, dried oregano, dried basil, salt, and pepper. Stir to combine.
3. Cover and cook on low for 6-8 hours or on high for 3-4 hours.
4. Cook the pasta according to package instructions until al dente. Drain.

5. Serve the beefy Bolognese sauce over
    the cooked pasta.

Nutrition per Serving:

❖ Calories: 420
❖ Fat: 18g
❖ Carbohydrates: 38g
❖ Protein: 28g

Mediterranean Quinoa Bowl

Ingredients:

1. 1 cup quinoa, rinsed
2. 2 cups vegetable broth
3. 1 can (15 ounces) chickpeas, drained and rinsed
4. 1 cup cherry tomatoes, halved
5. 1 cucumber, diced
6. 1/2 cup Kalamata olives, sliced
7. 1/4 cup red onion, finely chopped
8. 1/4 cup fresh parsley, chopped
9. 2 tablespoons olive oil
10. 2 tablespoons lemon juice
11. Salt and pepper to taste
12. Optional: crumbled feta cheese for topping

Instructions:

1. In the crockpot, combine quinoa and vegetable broth. Stir to combine.
2. Add chickpeas, cherry tomatoes, cucumber, Kalamata olives, red onion, and parsley to the quinoa mixture.

3. Drizzle olive oil and lemon juice over the ingredients. Season with salt and pepper. Stir well.
4. Cover and cook on low for 2-3 hours or until quinoa is cooked and the flavors have melded together.
5. Serve the Mediterranean quinoa in bowls, optionally topping with crumbled feta cheese.

Nutrition per Serving:

❖ Calories: 320
❖ Fat: 12g
❖ Carbohydrates: 45g
❖ Protein: 10g

Chapter 4

Flavorful International Dishes

Chicken Tikka Masala

Ingredients:

1. 1.5 lbs (680g) boneless, skinless chicken thighs, cut into bite-sized pieces
2. 1 cup plain Greek yogurt
3. 2 tablespoons lemon juice
4. 2 tablespoons olive oil
5. 2 cloves garlic, minced
6. 1 tablespoon grated ginger
7. 2 teaspoons ground cumin
8. 2 teaspoons paprika
9. 2 teaspoons ground turmeric
10. 1 teaspoon ground coriander
11. 1 teaspoon garam masala
12. 1/2 teaspoon cayenne pepper
13. Salt and black pepper to taste
14. 1 onion, finely chopped
15. 1 can (14 oz) crushed tomatoes

16.1 cup heavy cream

17.Fresh cilantro for garnish

Instructions:

1. In a bowl, combine yogurt, lemon juice, olive oil, garlic, ginger, cumin, paprika, turmeric, coriander, garam masala, cayenne pepper, salt, and black pepper. Mix well.
2. Add the chicken pieces to the marinade, ensuring they are coated thoroughly. Cover and refrigerate for at least 1 hour or overnight.
3. In a slow cooker, place the marinated chicken, chopped onion, and crushed tomatoes. Stir to combine.
4. Cover and cook on low heat for 6 hours.
5. Stir in the heavy cream and let it cook for an additional 30 minutes.
6. Serve hot, garnished with fresh cilantro. Enjoy with rice or naan bread.

Nutrition per serving:

❖ Calories: 380
❖ Protein: 28g
❖ Fat: 25g
❖ Carbohydrates: 10g
❖ Fiber: 2g
❖ Sugar: 5g
❖ Sodium: 320mg

Mexican Beef Carnitas

Ingredients:

1. 2 lbs (900g) beef chuck roast, cut into chunks
2. 1 tablespoon olive oil
3. 1 onion, diced
4. 4 cloves garlic, minced
5. 1 can (4 oz) diced green chilies
6. 1 teaspoon ground cumin
7. 1 teaspoon smoked paprika
8. 1 teaspoon dried oregano
9. 1/2 teaspoon chili powder
10. Salt and black pepper to taste
11. 1/2 cup beef broth
12. Juice of 1 lime
13. Fresh cilantro for garnish
14. Corn tortillas, for serving

Instructions:

1. Heat olive oil in a skillet over medium-high heat. Brown the beef chunks on all sides. Transfer the browned beef to the slow cooker.

2. In the same skillet, sauté onions and garlic until soft. Add diced green chilies, cumin, paprika, oregano, chili powder, salt, and black pepper. Cook for 2 minutes.
3. Pour the onion and spice mixture over the beef in the slow cooker. Add beef broth and lime juice.
4. Cover and cook on low heat for 6-8 hours or until the beef is tender and easily shredded.
5. Shred the beef using two forks. Serve the carnitas in corn tortillas, garnished with fresh cilantro.

Nutrition per serving:

- ❖ Calories: 280
- ❖ Protein: 26g
- ❖ Fat: 18g
- ❖ Carbohydrates: 5g
- ❖ Fiber: 1g
- ❖ Sugar: 1g
- ❖ Sodium: 280mg

Thai Red Curry

Ingredients:

1. 1 lb (450g) boneless, skinless chicken breast, thinly sliced
2. 1 can (14 oz) coconut milk
3. 2 tablespoons red curry paste
4. 1 red bell pepper, sliced
5. 1 yellow bell pepper, sliced
6. 1 cup sliced mushrooms
7. 1 small eggplant, diced
8. 1 tablespoon fish sauce
9. 1 tablespoon brown sugar
10. Juice of 1 lime
11. Fresh basil leaves for garnish
12. Cooked jasmine rice, for serving

Instructions:

1. In the slow cooker, combine coconut milk and red curry paste. Mix until well combined.
2. Add chicken slices, red bell pepper, yellow bell pepper, mushrooms, and diced eggplant to the slow cooker. Stir to coat with the curry mixture.

3. Cover and cook on low heat for 4 hours or until the chicken is cooked through and the vegetables are tender.
4. Stir in fish sauce, brown sugar, and lime juice. Let it cook for an additional 15 minutes.
5. Serve hot over jasmine rice, garnished with fresh basil leaves.

Nutrition per serving:

- ❖ Calories: 320
- ❖ Protein: 24g
- ❖ Fat: 20g
- ❖ Carbohydrates: 12g
- ❖ Fiber: 4g
- ❖ Sugar: 6g
- ❖ Sodium: 540mg

Chapter 5

Healthy Vegetarian Options

Lentil and Vegetable Curry

Ingredients:

1. 1 cup dried lentils, rinsed
2. 2 cups vegetable broth
3. 1 tablespoon olive oil
4. 1 onion, diced
5. 3 cloves garlic, minced
6. 1 tablespoon curry powder
7. 1 teaspoon ground turmeric
8. 1 can (14 oz) diced tomatoes
9. 2 cups mixed vegetables (such as bell peppers, carrots, and peas)
10. Salt and pepper to taste
11. Fresh cilantro for garnish (optional)

Instructions:

1. In a pot, combine lentils and vegetable broth. Bring to a boil, then

reduce heat and simmer for 15-20 minutes until lentils are tender.

2. In a separate pan, heat olive oil over medium heat. Add diced onion and cook until translucent. Add garlic, curry powder, and turmeric, stirring for another minute.

3. Add the onion-spice mixture to the pot of lentils. Stir in the diced tomatoes and mixed vegetables. Simmer for an additional 10-15 minutes.

4. Season with salt and pepper to taste. Garnish with fresh cilantro if desired. Serve hot over rice or with naan bread.

Nutrition per Serving (approximate):

Calories: 250 | Total Fat: 4g | Carbohydrates: 40g | Fiber: 15g | Protein: 15g

Ratatouille

Ingredients:

1. 1 eggplant, diced
2. 2 zucchinis, diced
3. 1 bell pepper, diced
4. 1 onion, diced
5. 3 cloves garlic, minced
6. 2 tomatoes, diced
7. 2 tablespoons olive oil
8. 1 teaspoon dried thyme
9. 1 teaspoon dried basil
10. Salt and pepper to taste
11. Fresh basil for garnish (optional)

Instructions:

1. Preheat the oven to 375°F (190°C).
2. In a baking dish, combine all diced vegetables and minced garlic. Drizzle with olive oil and sprinkle with dried thyme, dried basil, salt, and pepper. Toss to coat evenly.
3. Cover the baking dish with foil and bake for 45 minutes. Remove the foil and bake for an additional 15-20

minutes until vegetables are tender and slightly caramelized.

4. Garnish with fresh basil if desired. Serve as a side dish or over cooked quinoa or pasta.

Nutrition per Serving (approximate):

Calories: 120 | Total Fat: 7g | Carbohydrates: 15g | Fiber: 6g | Protein: 3g

Veggie-Packed Minestrone

Ingredients:

1. 1 tablespoon olive oil
2. 1 onion, diced
3. 2 carrots, diced
4. 2 celery stalks, diced
5. 3 cloves garlic, minced
6. 1 can (14 oz) diced tomatoes
7. 6 cups vegetable broth
8. 1 can (15 oz) kidney beans, drained and rinsed
9. 1 cup small pasta (such as ditalini or elbow)
10. 2 cups chopped spinach or kale
11. 1 teaspoon dried oregano
12. Salt and pepper to taste
13. Grated Parmesan cheese for garnish (optional)

Instructions:

1. In a large pot, heat olive oil over medium heat. Add diced onion, carrots, celery, and garlic. Cook until softened, about 5-7 minutes.

2. Stir in diced tomatoes, vegetable broth, kidney beans, pasta, and dried oregano. Bring to a boil, then reduce heat and simmer for 15-20 minutes until pasta is cooked.
3. Add chopped spinach or kale to the pot and cook for an additional 5 minutes until wilted. Season with salt and pepper to taste.
4. Serve hot, garnished with grated Parmesan cheese if desired.

Nutrition per Serving (approximate):

Calories: 220 | Total Fat: 4g | Carbohydrates: 38g | Fiber: 8g | Protein: 9g

Chapter 6

Sweet Treats and Desserts

Slow Cooker Apple Crisp
Ingredients:

1. 6 cups of peeled and sliced apples
2. 1 cup rolled oats
3. 1/2 cup all-purpose flour
4. 1/2 cup brown sugar
5. 1 teaspoon cinnamon
6. 1/2 teaspoon nutmeg
7. 1/2 cup unsalted butter, melted
8. Vanilla ice cream or whipped cream (optional, for serving)

Instructions:

1. Grease the inside of the slow cooker.
2. Place the sliced apples at the bottom of the slow cooker.
3. In a separate bowl, mix rolled oats, flour, brown sugar, cinnamon,

nutmeg, and melted butter until crumbly.

4. Spread this mixture evenly over the apples in the slow cooker.
5. Cover and cook on low for 4-5 hours until the apples are tender.
6. Serve warm, topped with a scoop of vanilla ice cream or a dollop of whipped cream if desired.

Nutrition per Serving (without toppings):

- ❖ Calories: 240
- ❖ Fat: 10g
- ❖ Carbohydrates: 38g
- ❖ Fiber: 5g
- ❖ Protein: 2g

Chocolate Lava Cake

Ingredients:

1. 1 cup semi-sweet chocolate chips
2. 1/2 cup unsalted butter
3. 1/4 cup granulated sugar
4. 2 large eggs
5. 2 teaspoons vanilla extract
6. 1/4 cup all-purpose flour
7. Pinch of salt
8. Vanilla ice cream or powdered sugar (optional, for serving)

Instructions:

1. Grease the inside of the slow cooker.
2. In a microwave-safe bowl, melt the chocolate chips and butter together, stirring until smooth.
3. Stir in sugar, eggs, and vanilla extract until well combined.
4. Add flour and a pinch of salt, mix until just combined.
5. Pour the batter into the slow cooker.

6. Cover and cook on low for 2-3 hours. The edges should be set, but the center will remain slightly gooey.
7. Serve warm with a scoop of vanilla ice cream or a dusting of powdered sugar if desired.

Nutrition per Serving (without toppings):

- ❖ Calories: 320
- ❖ Fat: 22g
- ❖ Carbohydrates: 28g
- ❖ Fiber: 2g
- ❖ Protein: 4g

Berry Bread Pudding

Ingredients:

1. 6 cups cubed bread (preferably day-old)
2. 2 cups mixed berries (strawberries, blueberries, raspberries)
3. 4 large eggs
4. 2 cups milk
5. 1/2 cup granulated sugar
6. 1 teaspoon vanilla extract
7. 1/2 teaspoon cinnamon
8. Whipped cream or berry sauce (optional, for serving)

Instructions:

1. Grease the inside of the slow cooker.
2. Place half of the cubed bread in the slow cooker, followed by half of the mixed berries. Repeat with the remaining bread and berries.
3. In a bowl, whisk together eggs, milk, sugar, vanilla extract, and cinnamon.
4. Pour this mixture evenly over the bread and berries in the slow cooker.

5. Cover and cook on low for 3-4 hours until the bread pudding is set and slightly golden on top.
6. Serve warm, optionally topped with whipped cream or a drizzle of berry sauce.

Nutrition per Serving (without toppings):

❖ Calories: 280
❖ Fat: 8g
❖ Carbohydrates: 45g
❖ Fiber: 4g
❖ Protein: 8g

More recipes to indulge

Chicken and Rice Casserole

Ingredients:

1. 1 ½ lbs chicken thighs, boneless, skinless
2. 1 cup long-grain white rice
3. 1 onion, finely chopped
4. 2 cups chicken broth
5. 1 cup frozen peas
6. 1 teaspoon paprika
7. Salt and pepper to taste

Instructions:

1. Place chicken thighs, rice, onion, and chicken broth in the crockpot.
2. Sprinkle with paprika, salt, and pepper.
3. Cook on low for 4 hours until chicken is cooked through and rice is tender.
4. Stir in frozen peas, cover, and cook for an additional 10 minutes.
5. Serve hot.

Nutrition per Serving:

Calories: 380 | Protein: 28g | Carbohydrates: 40g | Fat: 10g

Vegetarian Chili

Ingredients:

1. 2 cans (15 oz each) kidney beans, drained and rinsed
2. 1 can (28 oz) diced tomatoes
3. 1 onion, diced
4. 1 bell pepper, diced
5. 1 cup frozen corn
6. 2 cloves garlic, minced
7. 2 tablespoons chili powder
8. 1 teaspoon cumin
9. Salt and pepper to taste

Instructions:

1. Combine all ingredients in the crockpot.
2. Stir well, ensuring everything is mixed.
3. Cook on low for 6-8 hours or high for 3-4 hours.

4. Serve with your choice of toppings.

Nutrition per Serving:

Calories: 290 | Protein: 15g | Carbohydrates: 55g | Fat: 2g

Lemon Garlic Chicken

Ingredients:

1. 4 chicken breasts, boneless, skinless
2. ½ cup chicken broth
3. 3 cloves garlic, minced
4. Zest and juice of 1 lemon
5. 1 teaspoon dried thyme
6. Salt and pepper to taste
7. Fresh parsley for garnish (optional)

Instructions:

1. Place chicken breasts in the crockpot.
2. In a bowl, mix chicken broth, garlic, lemon zest, lemon juice, thyme, salt, and pepper.
3. Pour the mixture over the chicken.
4. Cook on low for 4-5 hours until chicken is tender.

5. Garnish with fresh parsley before serving.

Nutrition per Serving:

Calories: 220 | Protein: 35g | Carbohydrates: 2g | Fat: 7g

Beef and Broccoli

Ingredients:

1. 1 ½ lbs beef sirloin, thinly sliced
2. 1 cup beef broth
3. ⅓ cup soy sauce
4. 3 cloves garlic, minced
5. 2 tablespoons honey
6. 1 teaspoon ginger, grated
7. 2 cups broccoli florets
8. 2 tablespoons cornstarch
9. Sesame seeds for garnish (optional)

Instructions:

1. Place beef, beef broth, soy sauce, garlic, honey, and ginger in the crockpot. Mix well.
2. Cook on low for 4 hours.

3. Add broccoli to the crockpot and cook for an additional 30 minutes.
4. In a small bowl, mix cornstarch with 2 tablespoons of water. Stir into the crockpot to thicken the sauce.
5. Serve over rice, garnished with sesame seeds if desired.

Nutrition per Serving:

Calories: 320 | Protein: 40g | Carbohydrates: 15g | Fat: 10g

Creamy Mushroom and Spinach Pasta

Ingredients:

1. 8 oz pasta (penne or fusilli)
2. 2 cups mushrooms, sliced
3. 2 cloves garlic, minced
4. 2 cups fresh spinach
5. 2 cups vegetable broth
6. 1 cup heavy cream
7. ½ cup grated Parmesan cheese
8. Salt and pepper to taste

Instructions:

1. Place pasta, mushrooms, garlic, spinach, and vegetable broth in the crockpot.
2. Stir well and cook on low for 2-3 hours until pasta is tender.
3. Stir in heavy cream and Parmesan cheese.
4. Season with salt and pepper before serving.

Nutrition per Serving:

Calories: 450 | Protein: 15g | Carbohydrates: 45g | Fat: 25g

Crockpot Ratatouille

Ingredients:

1. 1 eggplant, diced
2. 2 zucchinis, sliced
3. 1 bell pepper, chopped
4. 1 onion, diced
5. 2 cloves garlic, minced
6. 2 cups diced tomatoes
7. 1 teaspoon dried basil
8. 1 teaspoon dried thyme
9. Salt and pepper to taste

Instructions:

1. Place eggplant, zucchinis, bell pepper, onion, garlic, and diced tomatoes in the crockpot.
2. Add dried basil, thyme, salt, and pepper. Mix well.
3. Cook on low for 4-6 hours until vegetables are tender.
4. Serve as a side dish or over cooked quinoa or rice.

Nutrition per Serving:

**Calories: 120 | Protein: 3g |
Carbohydrates: 25g | Fat: 1g**

Teriyaki Turkey Meatballs

Ingredients:

1. 1 lb ground turkey
2. 1 egg
3. ⅓ cup breadcrumbs
4. ½ cup soy sauce
5. ¼ cup honey
6. 2 cloves garlic, minced
7. 1 teaspoon ginger, grated
8. Green onions for garnish (optional)
9. Sesame seeds for garnish (optional)

Instructions:

1. In a bowl, combine ground turkey, egg, and breadcrumbs. Form into meatballs.
2. Place meatballs in the crockpot.
3. In another bowl, mix soy sauce, honey, garlic, and ginger. Pour over the meatballs.
4. Cook on low for 3-4 hours.

5. Garnish with green onions and sesame seeds before serving.

Nutrition per Serving:

Calories: 220 | Protein: 20g | Carbohydrates: 15g | Fat: 8g

Mediterranean Quinoa Stew

Ingredients:

1. 1 cup quinoa, rinsed
2. 2 cups vegetable broth
3. 1 can (15 oz) chickpeas, drained and rinsed
4. 1 cup diced tomatoes
5. 1 bell pepper, diced
6. 1 zucchini, diced
7. 2 teaspoons dried oregano
8. Salt and pepper to taste
9. Fresh parsley for garnish (optional)

Instructions:

1. Place quinoa, vegetable broth, chickpeas, diced tomatoes, bell

pepper, zucchini, oregano, salt, and pepper in the crockpot.

2. Stir well and cook on low for 2-3 hours.

3. Garnish with fresh parsley before serving.

Nutrition per Serving:

Calories: 280 | Protein: 12g | Carbohydrates: 50g | Fat: 4g

Lemon Herb Salmon

Ingredients:

1. 4 salmon fillets
2. Zest and juice of 1 lemon
3. 2 tablespoons olive oil
4. 2 cloves garlic, minced
5. 1 teaspoon dried dill
6. Salt and pepper to taste
7. Fresh dill for garnish (optional)

Instructions:

1. Place salmon fillets in the crockpot.

2. In a bowl, mix lemon zest, lemon juice, olive oil, garlic, dried dill, salt, and pepper. Pour over the salmon.
3. Cook on low for 1-2 hours until salmon flakes easily with a fork.
4. Garnish with fresh dill before serving.

Nutrition per Serving:

Calories: 300 | Protein: 25g | Carbohydrates: 2g | Fat: 20g

BBQ Pulled Pork Sandwiches

Ingredients:

1. 2 lbs pork shoulder, trimmed
2. 1 cup BBQ sauce
3. ½ cup apple cider vinegar
4. ¼ cup brown sugar
5. 1 tablespoon Worcestershire sauce
6. 1 teaspoon smoked paprika
7. Hamburger buns for serving
8. Coleslaw for topping (optional)

Instructions:

1. Place pork shoulder in the crockpot.
2. In a bowl, mix BBQ sauce, apple cider vinegar, brown sugar, Worcestershire sauce, and smoked paprika. Pour over the pork.
3. Cook on low for 8 hours or until the pork is tender and easily shreds.
4. Shred the pork using two forks.
5. Serve on hamburger buns, topped with coleslaw if desired.

Nutrition per Serving:

Calories: 380 | Protein: 25g | Carbohydrates: 30g | Fat: 18g

Creamy Chicken Alfredo Pasta
Ingredients:

1. 1 ½ lbs chicken breasts, diced
2. 2 cups chicken broth
3. 1 cup heavy cream
4. 1 cup grated Parmesan cheese
5. 8 oz fettuccine pasta
6. 2 cups broccoli florets
7. 2 cloves garlic, minced

8. Salt and pepper to taste

Instructions:

1. Place chicken, chicken broth, heavy cream, Parmesan cheese, fettuccine pasta, broccoli, and garlic in the crockpot.
2. Stir well and cook on low for 2-3 hours, stirring occasionally until the pasta is cooked and the sauce is creamy.
3. Season with salt and pepper before serving.

Nutrition per Serving:

Calories: 480 | Protein: 40g | Carbohydrates: 30g | Fat: 22g

Beef Burrito Bowls

Ingredients:

1. 1 ½ lbs beef sirloin, thinly sliced
2. 1 cup beef broth
3. 1 can (15 oz) black beans, drained and rinsed
4. 1 cup corn kernels
5. 1 bell pepper, diced
6. 1 onion, diced
7. 2 teaspoons chili powder
8. 1 teaspoon cumin
9. Salt and pepper to taste
10. Cooked rice for serving

Instructions:

1. Place beef, beef broth, black beans, corn, bell pepper, onion, chili powder, cumin, salt, and pepper in the crockpot.
2. Mix well and cook on low for 6-8 hours.
3. Serve over cooked rice.

Nutrition per Serving:

Calories: 420 | Protein: 35g | Carbohydrates: 40g | Fat: 15g

Mediterranean Chicken with Olives and Artichokes

Ingredients:

1. 1 ½ lbs chicken thighs, boneless, skinless
2. 1 can (14 oz) artichoke hearts, drained
3. ½ cup pitted Kalamata olives
4. 1 onion, sliced
5. 3 cloves garlic, minced
6. 1 teaspoon dried oregano
7. ½ teaspoon dried thyme
8. ½ cup chicken broth
9. Salt and pepper to taste
10. Fresh parsley for garnish (optional)

Instructions:

1. Place chicken thighs, artichoke hearts, olives, onion, garlic, oregano, thyme, chicken broth, salt, and pepper in the crockpot.

2. Mix well and cook on low for 4-5 hours until chicken is tender.
3. Garnish with fresh parsley before serving.

Nutrition per Serving:

Calories: 320 | Protein: 30g | Carbohydrates: 10g | Fat: 18g

Crockpot Beef and Vegetable Curry

Ingredients:

1. 1 ½ lbs beef stew meat, cubed
2. 1 can (14 oz) coconut milk
3. 1 onion, chopped
4. 2 cloves garlic, minced
5. 2 cups cauliflower florets
6. 1 cup carrots, sliced
7. 1 bell pepper, diced
8. 2 tablespoons curry powder
9. Salt and pepper to taste
10. Fresh cilantro for garnish (optional)

Instructions:

1. Place beef, coconut milk, onion, garlic, cauliflower, carrots, bell pepper, curry powder, salt, and pepper in the crockpot.
2. Stir well and cook on low for 6-8 hours until beef is tender.
3. Serve over rice and garnish with fresh cilantro if desired.

Nutrition per Serving:

Calories: 380 | Protein: 30g | Carbohydrates: 15g | Fat: 22g

Lemon Garlic Butter Shrimp

Ingredients:

1. 1 lb shrimp, peeled and deveined
2. ½ cup chicken broth
3. 4 tablespoons butter
4. 4 cloves garlic, minced
5. Zest and juice of 1 lemon
6. 1 teaspoon Italian seasoning
7. Salt and pepper to taste
8. Fresh parsley for garnish (optional)

Instructions:

1. Place shrimp, chicken broth, butter, garlic, lemon zest, lemon juice, Italian seasoning, salt, and pepper in the crockpot.
2. Cook on low for 1-2 hours until shrimp are pink and cooked through.
3. Garnish with fresh parsley before serving.

Nutrition per Serving:

Calories: 220 | Protein: 25g | Carbohydrates: 2g | Fat: 12g

Turkey and Sweet Potato Chili

Ingredients:

1. 1 lb ground turkey
2. 2 sweet potatoes, peeled and diced
3. 1 can (15 oz) kidney beans, drained and rinsed
4. 1 can (14 oz) diced tomatoes
5. 1 onion, diced
6. 2 cloves garlic, minced
7. 2 tablespoons chili powder
8. 1 teaspoon cumin

9. Salt and pepper to taste
10. Chopped cilantro for garnish (optional)

Instructions:

1. In a skillet, brown the ground turkey over medium heat until cooked through. Drain excess fat.
2. Place cooked turkey, sweet potatoes, kidney beans, diced tomatoes, onion, garlic, chili powder, cumin, salt, and pepper in the crockpot.
3. Stir well and cook on low for 6-8 hours.
4. Garnish with chopped cilantro before serving.

Nutrition per Serving:

Calories: 320 | Protein: 25g | Carbohydrates: 35g | Fat: 10g

Hawaiian Pineapple Chicken

Ingredients:

1. 1 ½ lbs chicken thighs, boneless, skinless
2. 1 can (20 oz) pineapple chunks, drained (reserve juice)
3. ½ cup pineapple juice
4. ⅓ cup soy sauce
5. ¼ cup brown sugar
6. 2 tablespoons ketchup
7. 2 cloves garlic, minced
8. 1 teaspoon ginger, grated
9. 1 bell pepper, diced
10. 1 onion, diced
11. Cooked rice for serving

Instructions:

1. Place chicken thighs, pineapple chunks, pineapple juice, soy sauce, brown sugar, ketchup, garlic, ginger, bell pepper, and onion in the crockpot.
2. Mix well and cook on low for 4-5 hours until chicken is tender.

3. Serve over cooked rice.

Nutrition per Serving:

Calories: 380 | Protein: 30g | Carbohydrates: 40g | Fat: 10g

Creamy Mushroom Chicken

Ingredients:

1. 1 ½ lbs chicken breasts, boneless, skinless
2. 2 cups mushrooms, sliced
3. 1 onion, finely chopped
4. 2 cloves garlic, minced
5. 1 cup chicken broth
6. 1 cup heavy cream
7. 2 tablespoons flour
8. 2 tablespoons butter
9. Salt and pepper to taste
10. Chopped parsley for garnish (optional)

Instructions:

1. Season chicken breasts with salt and pepper and place them in the crockpot.
2. In a skillet, melt butter and sauté mushrooms, onion, and garlic until soft.
3. Sprinkle flour over the mushroom mixture and cook for 1-2 minutes.
4. Transfer the mushroom mixture to the crockpot with the chicken.
5. Pour in chicken broth and cook on low for 3-4 hours.
6. Stir in heavy cream and cook for an additional 30 minutes.
7. Garnish with chopped parsley before serving.

Nutrition per Serving:

Calories: 320 | Protein: 30g | Carbohydrates: 10g | Fat: 18g

Conclusion

We have set out on a mission to balance the art of nutritional meals with hectic schedules along this culinary journey. The goal at the start of the trip was to combine convenience with nutrition. This cookbook is the result of a combination of the author's own experience and her knowledge as a nutritionist and a man navigating the turbulent waves of time restrictions.

The recipes on these pages represent a dedication to tasty, healthful meals that respect time limits; they are more than simply lists of ingredients and directions. Every meal is carefully planned and assembled to exude a sense of comfort, flavor, and well-being.

These recipes, which range from robust stews to enticing ethnic tastes and quick, delicious pasta dishes, invite men—those balancing hectic schedules and demanding careers—to rediscover the pleasure of cooking at home. Our faithful companion in our culinary adventure, the crockpot, is a source of convenience that turns ordinary items into delectable treats.

This cookbook is leaving a trail of delicious smells, warm memories, and a reminder that food does not have to give way to life's inexorable speed. It's a celebration of the pleasure of cooking, the satisfaction that comes from a full stomach, and the power that comes from giving our bodies healthy, nourishing food.

I hope that these recipes bring you warmth, plenty, and the delight of thoughtful, delicious meals for the rest of your life.